For more information . . .

This booklet is only one of many free booklets for people with cancer. Here are some others you and your loved ones may find useful:

- *Biological Therapy: Treatments That Use Your Immune System To Fight Cancer*

- *Chemotherapy and You*

- *Eating Hints Before, During, and After Cancer Treatment*

- *Taking Part in Cancer Treatment Research Studies*

- *Pain Control*

- *Radiation Therapy and You*

- *Taking Time*

- *Thinking About Complementary and Alternative Medicine*

- *When Your Parent Has Cancer: A Guide for Teens*

- *When Someone You Love Is Being Treated for Cancer*

- *When Someone You Love Has Advanced Cancer*

These booklets are available from the National Cancer Institute (NCI.) To learn more about the specific type of cancer you have or to request any of these booklets, visit NCI's Web site (www.cancer.gov). You can also call NCI's Cancer Information Service at 1-800-4-CANCER (1-800-422-6237) to speak with an information specialist.

When Cancer Returns

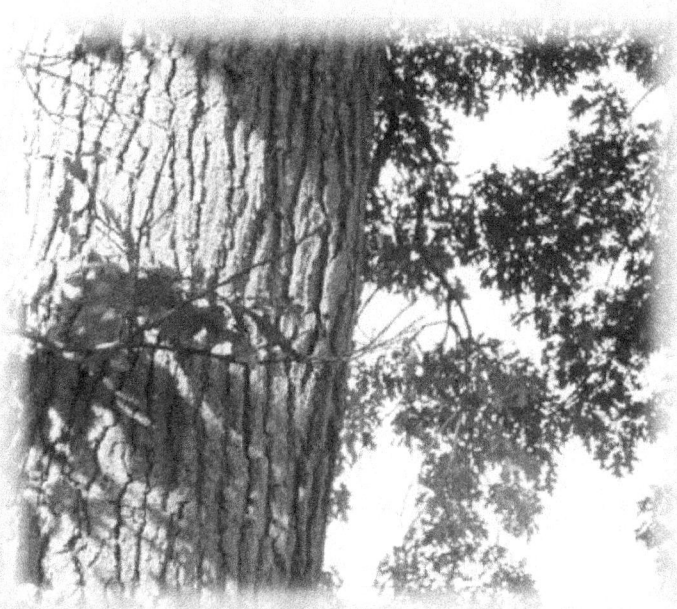

"When I found out I had cancer again,
I just felt numb. It was hard for me
to accept the news at first.
After a few weeks, though, I started
to really look at all my options
and things I could do for myself.
By doing this, it gave me back
some control."

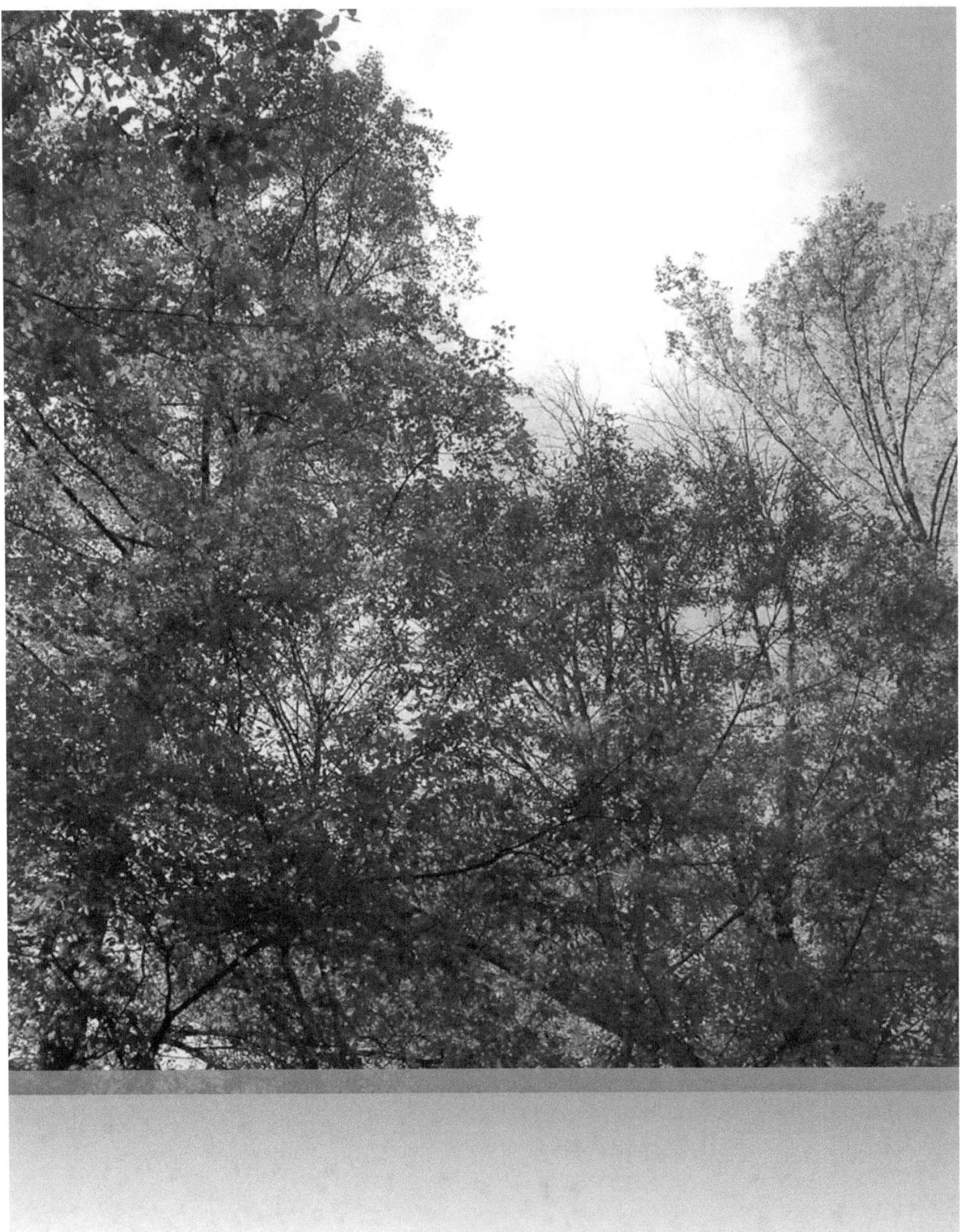

Table of Contents

Words that appear in **bold** in the text are defined in the
Words To Know section on page 34.

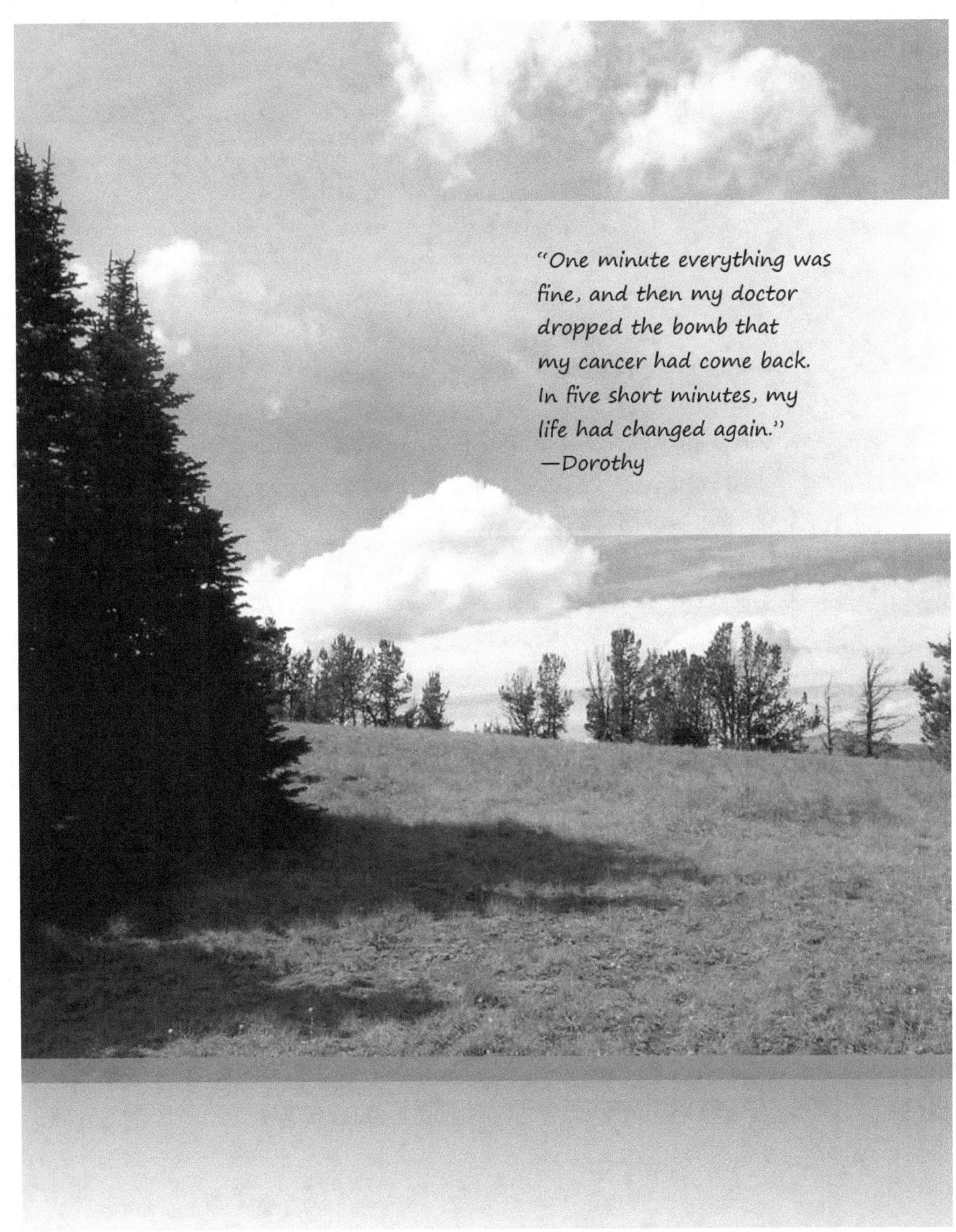

"One minute everything was fine, and then my doctor dropped the bomb that my cancer had come back. In five short minutes, my life had changed again."
—Dorothy

CHAPTER 1

Adjusting to the News

Maybe in the back of your mind, you feared that your **cancer** might return. Now you might be thinking, "How can this be happening to me again? Haven't I been through enough?"

You may be feeling shocked, angry, sad, or scared. Many people have these feelings. But you have something now that you didn't have before—experience. You've lived through cancer once. You know a lot about what to expect and hope for.

Also remember that treatments may have improved since you had your first cancer. New drugs or methods may help with your treatment or in managing side effects. In fact, cancer is now often thought of as a chronic disease, one which people manage for many years.

Using This Booklet

This booklet offers some general advice as you adjust to the news that your cancer has returned. It covers all aspects of your treatment. These include managing side effects and symptoms, as well as seeking emotional support.

Above all else, remember that your feelings count. There is no "right" way to cope. Some people need a lot of information. Others like a little at a time. Likewise, some sections in this booklet may address your needs. Others may not.

- Flip through the Table of Contents to look for topics you need.

- Using this guide along with those booklets listed on the inside front cover may help you find the information that you need.

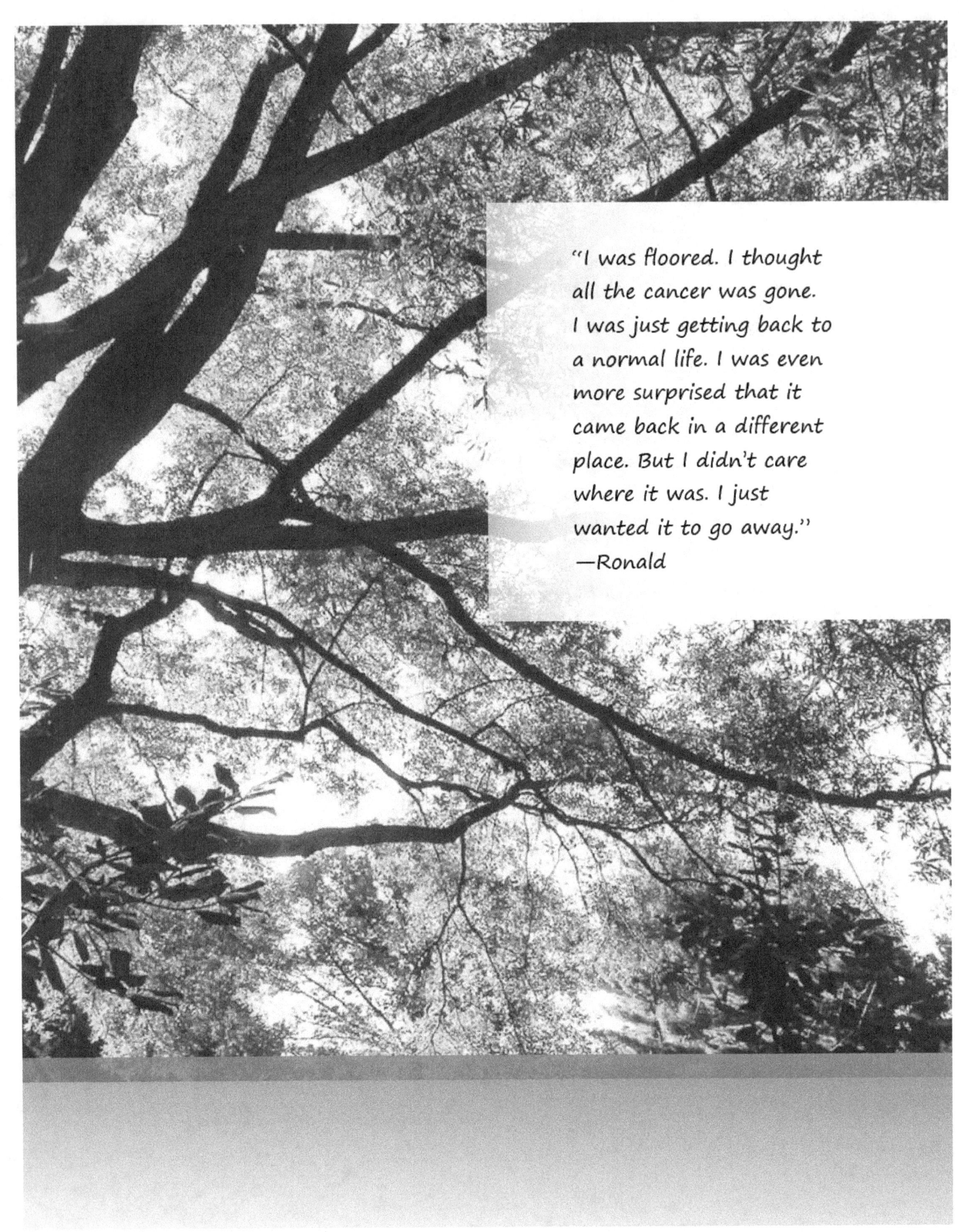

"I was floored. I thought all the cancer was gone. I was just getting back to a normal life. I was even more surprised that it came back in a different place. But I didn't care where it was. I just wanted it to go away."
—Ronald

CHAPTER 2

Why and Where Cancer Returns

When cancer comes back, doctors call it a **recurrence** (or **recurrent cancer**). Some things you should know are:

- A recurrent cancer starts with cancer cells that the first treatment didn't fully remove or destroy. Some may have been too small to be seen in follow-up. This doesn't mean that the treatment you received was wrong. And it doesn't mean that you did anything wrong, either. It just means that a small number of cancer cells survived the treatment. These cells grew over time into **tumors** or cancer that your doctor can now detect.

- When cancer comes back, it doesn't always show up in the same part of the body. For example, if you had colon cancer, it may come back in your liver. But the cancer is still called colon cancer. When the original cancer spreads to a new place, it is called a **metastasis** (meh-TAS-tuh-sis).

- It is possible to develop a completely new cancer that has nothing to do with your original cancer. But this doesn't happen very often. Recurrences are more common.

Where Cancer Can Return

Doctors define recurrent cancers by where they develop. The different types of recurrence are:

- **Local recurrence.** This means that the cancer is in the same place as the original cancer or is very close to it.

- **Regional recurrence.** This is when tumors grow in lymph nodes or tissues near the place of the original cancer.

- **Distant recurrence.** In these cases, the cancer has spread (metastasized) to organs or tissues far from the place of the original cancer.

Local cancer may be easier to treat than **regional** or **distant cancer**. But this can be different for each patient. Talk with your doctor about your options.

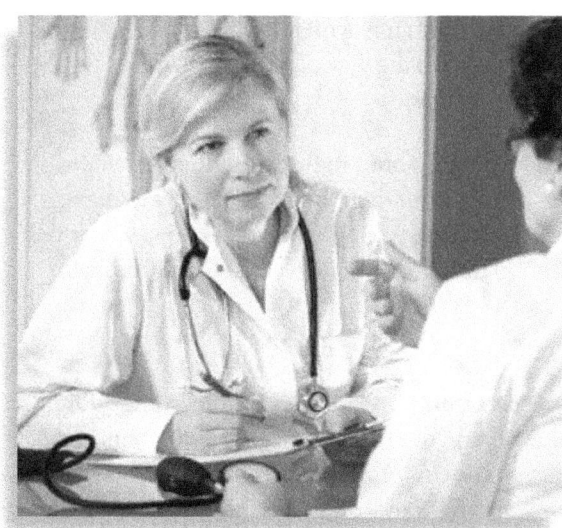

CHAPTER 3

Taking Control: Your Care and Treatment

Cancer that returns can affect all parts of your life. You may feel weak and no longer in control. But you don't have to feel that way. You can take part in your care and in making decisions. You can also talk with your health care team and loved ones as you decide about your care. This may help you feel a sense of control and well-being.

Talking With Your Health Care Team

"I always ask lots of questions because I want to be ready just in case something happens. I really do believe that everyone taking care of me has my best interests at heart. But I worry that if I don't ask about everything, they may forget to give me the answers." —Bonita

Many people have a treatment team of health providers who work together to help them. This team may include doctors, nurses, **oncology social workers**, **dietitians**, or other **specialists**. Some people don't like to ask about treatment choices or side effects. They think that doctors don't like being questioned. But this is not true. Most doctors want their patients to be involved in their own care. They want patients to discuss concerns with them.

Here are a few topics you may want to discuss with your health care team:

■ **Pain or Other Symptoms.** Be honest and open about how you feel. Tell your doctors if you have pain and where. Tell them what you expect in the way of pain relief. (See Chapter 4 for more about pain and other symptoms.)

■ **Communication.** Some people want to know details about their care. Others prefer to know as little as possible. Some people with cancer want their family members to make most of their decisions. What would you prefer? Decide what you want to know, how much you want to know, and when you've heard enough. Choose what is most comfortable for you. Then tell your doctor and family members. Ask that they follow through with your wishes.

■ **Family Wishes.** Some family members may have trouble dealing with cancer. They don't want to know how far the disease has advanced. Find out from your family members how much they want to know. And be sure to tell your doctors and nurses. Do this as soon as possible. It will help avoid conflicts or distress among your loved ones. (See page 27 to read more about talking with your loved ones.)

Other Tips for Talking With Your Health Care Team

"You need a notebook because you go to the doctors and they're telling you things, and you're so scared that you don't really listen. Then you get home, and you can't even remember what they said." —Jake

■ Speak openly about your needs, questions, and concerns. Don't be embarrassed to ask your doctor to repeat or explain something.

■ Keep a file or notebook of all the papers and test results that your doctor has given you. Take this file to your visits. Also keep records or a diary of all your visits. List the drugs and tests you have taken. Then you can refer to your records when you need to. Many patients say this is helpful, especially when you meet with a new doctor for the first time.

■ Write down your questions before you see your doctors so you will remember them. (See the box on page 10.)

■ Ask a family member or friend to go to the doctor's office with you. They can help you ask questions to get a clear sense of what to expect. This can be an emotional time. You may have trouble focusing on what the doctor says. It may be easier for someone else to take notes. Then you can review them later.

■ Ask your doctor if it's okay to tape-record your talks.

■ Tell your doctor if you want to get dressed before talking about your results. Wearing a gown or robe is distracting for some patients. They find it harder to focus on what the doctor is saying.

Treatment Choices

There are many treatment choices for recurrent cancer. Your treatment will depend partly on the type of cancer and the treatment you had before. It will also depend on where the cancer has recurred. For example:

■ A local recurrence may be best treated by **surgery** or **radiation therapy**. This means that the doctor removes the tumor or destroys it with radiation.

■ A distant recurrence may need **chemotherapy**, **biological therapy**, or radiation therapy. (For more information see the NCI booklets *Radiation Therapy and You,* Chemotherapy *and You*, and *Biological Therapy*.)

It's important to ask your doctor questions about all your treatment choices. You may want to get a **second opinion** as well. You may also want to ask whether a **clinical trial** is an option for you.

Should I Get A Second Opinion?

Some patients worry that doctors will be offended if they ask for a second opinion. Usually the opposite is true. Most doctors welcome a second opinion. And many health insurance companies will pay for them.

If you get a second opinion, the doctor may agree with your first doctor's treatment plan. Or the second doctor may suggest another approach. Either way, you have more information and perhaps a greater sense of control. You can feel more confident about the decisions you make, knowing that you've looked at your options.

Decide on the most important things you need to ask your doctor or nurse. Some ideas:

- What are my treatment choices?

- Which do you suggest for me?

- How is this treatment the same as or different from my last treatment?

- How successful is the treatment you recommend? Why is it best for me?

- Will I still be able to do things I enjoy with the treatment? Without the treatment?

- How long will I be on this treatment?

- Will I have side effects? If so, how long will they last?

- How can I manage the side effects?

- Will I have to stay in the hospital?

- Is a clinical trial available to me?

- Will I have to pay any costs in a clinical trial?

- If the treatment doesn't work, then what will I do?

Clinical Trials

Treatment clinical trials are research studies that try to find better ways to treat cancer. Every day, cancer researchers learn more about treatment options from clinical trials.

Each study has rules about who can take part. These rules include the person's age and type of cancer. They also cover earlier treatments and where the cancer has returned.

Clinical trials have both benefits and risks. Your doctor should tell you about them before you make any decisions about taking part.

There are different phases of clinical trials. They include:

- Phase I trials test what dose of a treatment is safe and how it should be given.

- Phase II trials discover how cancer responds to a new drug or treatment.

- Phase III trials compare an accepted cancer treatment (**standard treatment**) with a new treatment that researchers hope is better.

Taking part in a clinical trial could help you and others who get cancer in the future. But insurance and managed care plans do not always cover the costs. What they cover varies by plan and by study. If you want to learn more about clinical trials, talk with your health care team.

For more information about clinical trials, see NCI's brochure *Taking Part in Cancer Treatment Research Studies.*

Making Your Wishes Known

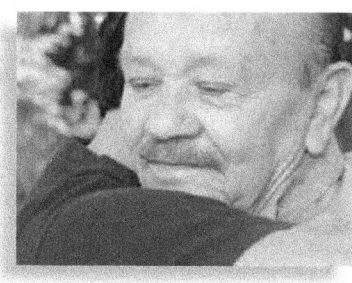

When cancer returns, the treatment goals may change, or they may be the same as they were for your first cancer. But for many people, it's the second cancer **diagnosis** that finally prompts them to make their wishes known. Although it can be tough to think about, and maybe even tougher to talk about, having recurrent cancer may prompt you to make certain decisions about what you want done for you if you are unable to speak for yourself.

Everyone should make a **will** and talk about end-of-life choices with loved ones. This is one of the most important things you can do. Also, think about giving someone you trust some rights to make medical decisions for you. You give these rights through legal documents called **advance directives**. These papers tell your loved ones and doctors what to do if you can't tell them yourself. They let you decide ahead of time how you want to be treated. These papers may include a **living will** and a **durable power of attorney for health care**.

Setting up an advance directive is not the same as giving up. Making such decisions at this time keeps you in control. You are making your wishes known for all to follow. This can help you worry less about the future and live each day to the fullest.

It's hard to talk about these issues. But it often comforts family members to know what you want. And it saves them from having to bring up the subject themselves. You may also gain peace of mind. You are making these hard choices for yourself instead of leaving them to your loved ones.

Make copies of your advance directives. Give them to your family members, your health care team, and your hospital medical records department. That way, everyone will know your decisions.

Legal Papers At-A-Glance

Advance directives

- A **living will** lets people know what kind of medical care you want if you are unable to speak for yourself.

- A **durable power of attorney for health care** names a person to make medical decisions for you if you can't make them yourself. This person is called a **health care proxy**.

Other legal papers that are not part of the advance directives

- A **will** tells how you want to divide your money and property among your heirs. (Heirs are usually the family members who survive you. You may also name other people as heirs in your will.)

- **Power of attorney** appoints a person to make financial decisions for you when you can't make them yourself.

Note: You do not always need a lawyer present to fill out these papers. But you may need a **notary public.** Each state has its own laws about advance directives. Check with your lawyer or social worker about the laws in your state. (For more, see the Resources on page 37.)

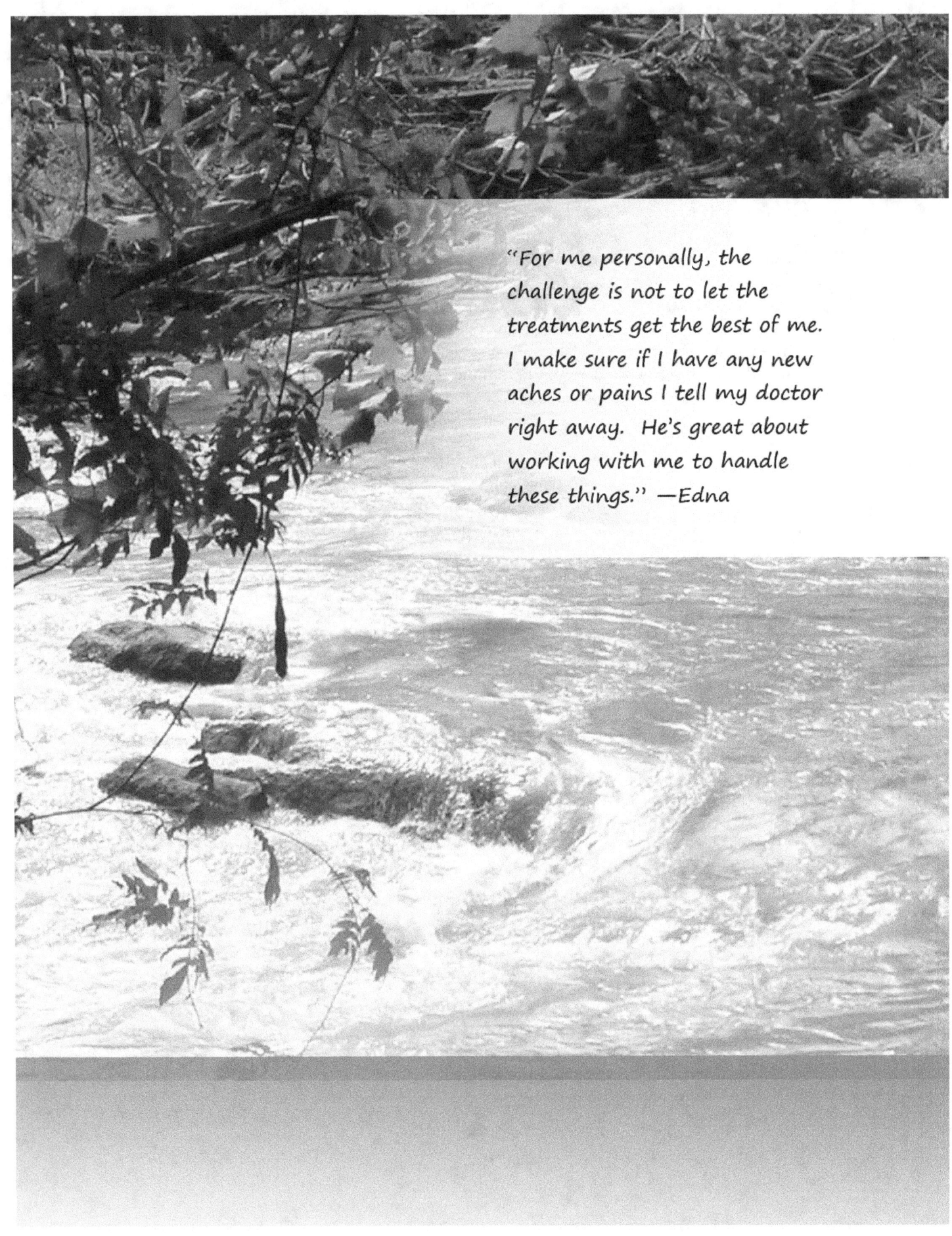

"For me personally, the challenge is not to let the treatments get the best of me. I make sure if I have any new aches or pains I tell my doctor right away. He's great about working with me to handle these things." —Edna

CHAPTER 4

Managing the Side Effects of Your Treatment

You probably already know about ways to manage the side effects of cancer treatment. If so, parts of this section will be a review for you. It outlines some of the support therapies cancer patients have found helpful.

For more information about side effects, see the NCI booklets *Radiation Therapy and You* and *Chemotherapy and You.*

Comfort Care

You have a right to comfort care both during and after treatment. This kind of care is often called **palliative** (PAL-ee-yuh-tiv) **care**. It includes treating or preventing cancer symptoms and the side effects caused by treatment. Comfort care can also mean getting help with emotional and spiritual problems during and after cancer treatment.

People once thought of palliative care as a way to comfort those dying of cancer. Doctors now offer this care to all cancer patients, beginning when the cancer is diagnosed. You should receive palliative care through treatment, survival, and advanced disease. Your **oncologist** may be able to help you. But a palliative care specialist may be the best person to treat some problems. Ask your doctor or nurse if there is a specialist you can go to.

Pain Control

Having cancer doesn't always mean that you'll have pain. But if you do, you shouldn't accept pain as normal. Your doctor can control pain with medicines and other treatments. Managing your pain helps you sleep and eat better. It makes it easier to enjoy your family and friends, and to focus on the things you enjoy.

Have regular talks with your health care team about your pain. Let them know what kind of pain it is, where it is, and how bad it is. These talks are important because pain can change throughout your illness. And your pain may show where cancer has returned after remission. Many hospitals have doctors who are experts in treating pain. Tell your doctor if you would like to talk to a pain specialist.

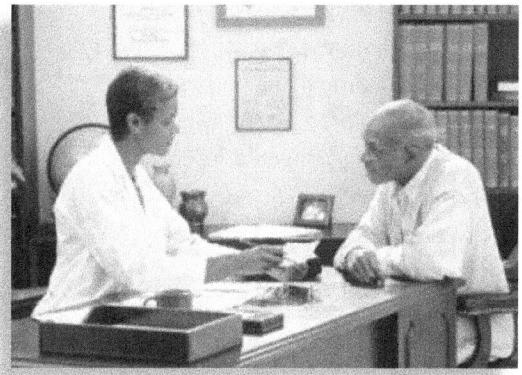

Controlling Pain

What To Tell Your Doctor

When describing pain to your doctor, give as much detail as you can. Your doctor may want to know:

- Where exactly is your pain? Does it move from one spot to another?

- How does the pain feel—dull, sharp, burning?

- How often do you have pain?

- How long does it last?

- Does it occur at a certain time of day—morning, afternoon, night?

- What makes the pain better?

- What makes it worse?

Using Strong Drugs To Control Pain

People with cancer often need strong medicine to help control their pain. Don't be afraid to ask for pain medicine or for larger doses if you need them. And the drugs will help you stay as comfortable as possible.

People with cancer hardly ever get addicted to these drugs. Sadly, fears of addiction sometimes prevent people from taking medicine for pain. The same fears also prompt family members to encourage loved ones to "hold off" between doses. But people in pain get the most relief when they take their medicines and treatments on a regular schedule.

Treatments can be used for all types of pain, including:

- Mild to medium pain

- Medium to very bad pain

- **Breakthrough pain**

- Tingling and burning pain

- Pain caused by swelling.

There are different ways to take pain medicine, such as:

- By mouth

- Through the skin (with a patch)

- By shots

- Through an I.V. pump.

Your medicine, and how you take it, will depend on the type of pain and its cause. For example, for constant pain you may need a steady dose of medicine over a long period of time. You might use a patch placed on the skin or a slow-release pill.

You may want to keep a pain diary to help you explain your pain to your doctor. In the diary, write down:

- The time of day you had the pain

- What you were doing when you felt the pain

- What it felt like

- Where you felt it.

Your doctor may also ask you some questions about how your pain affects your daily routine. Having your pain managed means that you can focus on living your life and not be distracted by pain.

To learn more, see the NCI booklet *Pain Control*.

Other Ways To Treat Pain

Cancer pain is usually treated with medicine and other therapies. But there are also some nondrug treatments. They are types of **complementary and alternative medicine (CAM)**.

Many people have found the methods listed below helpful. But talk with your health care team before trying any of them. Make sure they are safe and won't interfere with your cancer treatment.

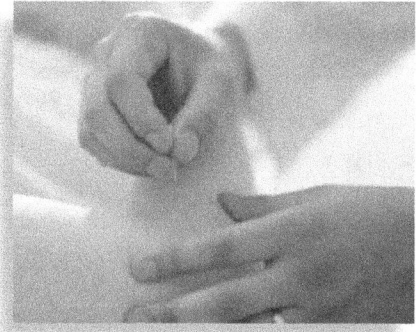

- **Acupuncture** is a form of Chinese medicine that stimulates certain points on the body using small needles. It may help treat nausea and control pain. Before using acupuncture, ask your health care team if it is safe for your type of cancer.

- **Imagery** is imagining scenes, pictures, or experiences to feel calmer or perhaps to help the body to heal.

- **Relaxation techniques** include deep breathing and exercises to relax your muscles.

- **Hypnosis** is a state of relaxed and focused attention. One focuses on a certain feeling, idea, or suggestion.

- **Biofeedback** is the use of a special machine to help the patient learn how to control certain body functions. These are things that we are normally not aware of (such as heart rate).

- **Massage therapy** brings relaxation and a sense of well-being by the gentle rubbing of different body parts or muscles. Before you try this, you need to check with your doctor. Massage is not recommended for some kinds of cancer.

These methods may also help manage stress. Again, talk to your health care team before using anything new, no matter how safe it may seem. Ask your health care team for more information about where to get these treatments. To learn more, see the NCI booklet *Thinking About Complementary and Alternative Medicine.*

Fatigue

Fatigue is more than feeling tired. Fatigue is exhaustion—not being able to do even the small things you used to do. A number of things can cause fatigue. Besides cancer treatment, they include anxiety, stress, and changes in your diet or sleeping patterns. If you are having some of these problems, you might want to:

■ Tell your doctor or nurse at your next visit. Ask about medicines that can help with fatigue.

■ Eat a well-balanced diet

■ Plan your days and do only what is important to you

■ Take short breaks every day to rest and relax

■ Take naps

■ Ask others for help.

Nausea and Vomiting

Nausea is feeling sick to your stomach. Vomiting means throwing up. Both can be a problem for cancer patients. Untreated nausea and vomiting can make you feel very tired. They can also make it hard to get treatments or to care for yourself. There are many drugs to help you control nausea and vomiting. Ask your doctor which medicines might work best for you.

You also may want to make these changes to your diet:

■ Eat small amounts of food five to six times a day.

■ Avoid foods that are sweet, fatty, salty, spicy, or have strong smells. These may make nausea and vomiting worse.

■ Have as much liquid as possible. You'll want to keep your body from getting too dry (dehydrated). Broth, ice cream, water, juices, herb teas, and watermelon are good choices.

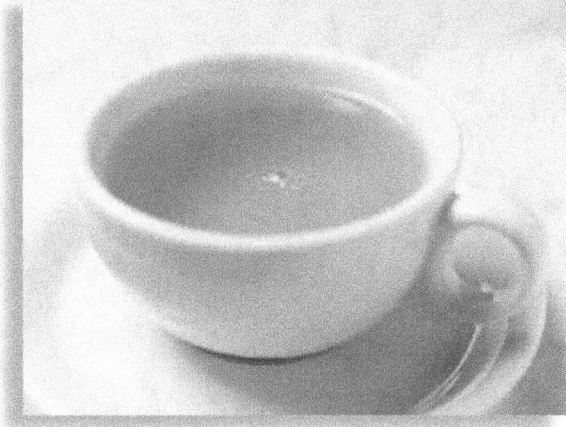

Nutrition

For some patients, it's hard to eat the foods they normally enjoy. For others, it's hard to eat anything at all. Are you having trouble eating or digesting food? If so, you may want to talk with your doctor about your diet. They may suggest:

- A special diet

- Other ways of getting the nutrition you need

- Tips on eating during treatment

- Seeing a dietitian.

For more information, see the NCI booklet *Eating Hints Before, During, and After Cancer Treatment.*

Sleep Problems

Illness, pain, stress, drugs, and being in the hospital can cause sleep problems. These problems may include:

- Having trouble falling asleep

- Sleeping only for short amounts of time

- Waking up in the middle of the night

- Having trouble getting back to sleep.

To help with your sleep problem, you may want to try:

- Reducing noise, dimming lights, making the room warmer or cooler, and using pillows to support your body

- Dressing in loose, soft clothing

- Going to the bathroom before bed

- Eating a high-protein snack 2 hours before bedtime (such as peanut butter, cheese, nuts, or some sliced chicken or turkey)

- Avoiding caffeine (coffee, tea, cola, hot cocoa)

- Keeping regular sleep hours

- Avoiding naps longer than 15-30 minutes

- Talking with your health care team about drugs to help you sleep.

Physical Therapy

Sometimes people with cancer feel pain in different parts of their body. Others feel weak and tired. And some feel stiffer than they used to. So it can become hard to move different body parts. If you are having any of these problems, your health care team may suggest you see a physical therapist. The therapist may use heat, cold, massage, pressure, or exercises to help you. Physical therapy may reduce tiredness and help your body function better. It may help with strength and balance as well. It also may help with stiffness and other side effects of radiation therapy.

Complementary and Alternative Medicine

Complementary and alternative medicine (CAM) treatment can be helpful for some people. And some CAM treatments are safe, such as those listed for pain on p. 11. But you may have read about different diets, vitamins, and herbs for treating your cancer or symptoms. Talk with your health care team before you try anything new. Here's why:

■ Some CAM treatments are not proven to work and could actually harm you.

■ You may have a dangerous reaction. Or the CAM treatment could interfere with the medicine your doctor has prescribed.

■ A "natural" product doesn't mean that it's a safe product.

Seek information about CAM treatments from trusted sources. Federal agencies and nonprofit cancer groups are good sources. You might also want to read the NCI booklet *Thinking About Complementary* and *Alternative Medicine:* or go to NCI's Office of Complementary and Alternative Medicine (www.cancer.gov/cam).

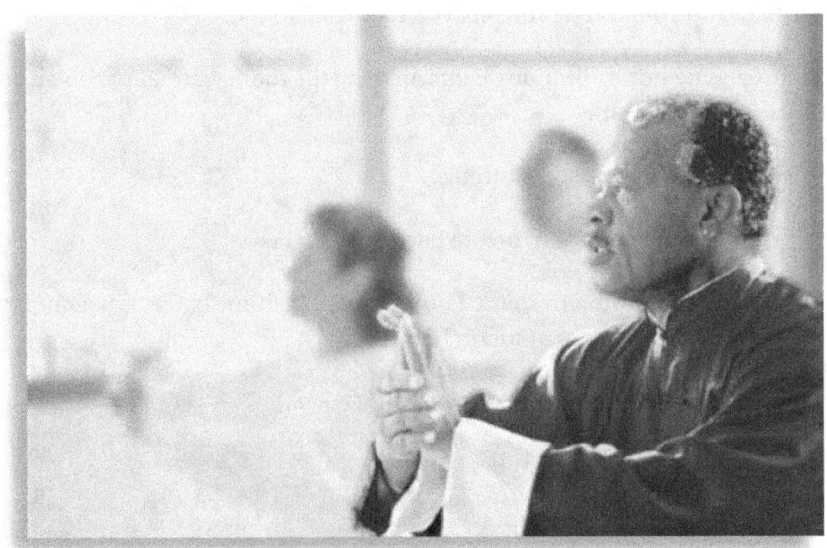

CHAPTER 5

Your Feelings

"Life has changed again and I can't help feeling frustrated with all that's going on. One minute I'll be upset and angry. Then the next minute, I'll start crying all of a sudden. I just never know what's coming next." —Kathy

People feel so many emotions when they find out that their cancer has come back. Shock, fear, anger, and denial are just a few. The new diagnosis hits them as hard as it did the first time, or even harder.

Regardless of your first reaction, starting cancer treatment again can place even more demands on your mind and spirit. You'll have good days and bad days. So just remember that it's okay to feel a lot of different emotions.

Some of these emotions may be ones you have had at other times in your life. But you may be feeling them more intensely. If you have dealt with them in the past, you may be able to cope with them now, too. If some of the feelings are new, or are so strong that it is hard to get through everyday activities, you may want to ask for help.

There are many people who may be able to help you. These include **health psychologists**, oncology social workers, other mental health experts, and leaders in your faith or spiritual community. They know many ways to help you cope with your feelings. See the section on page 21 for other ideas on how to cope.

Stress

"Once you get diagnosed again and go through more surgeries or procedures, your life is not normal. It's always in the back of your mind. What now? What's next?" —Margaret

Stress is a normal reaction to cancer. After all, you're dealing with a lot: treatment, family, your job, money, and day-to-day living. Sometimes, you may not even notice that you are stressed. But your family and friends probably see a change.

Anything that makes you feel calm or relaxed may help. So try to think of things that relax you and that you enjoy doing. Some people try deep breathing, listening to tapes that have nature sounds, or listening to music. See page 22 for more ideas on how to relieve stress.

Hope

"I just keep telling myself, 'You've got to have hope, you've got to have faith, because anything can happen.'" —Phil

While you may be sad or depressed about your cancer recurrence, you do have reasons to feel hopeful. Science has advanced and cancer treatments have improved. So more people are surviving cancer than ever before. Nearly 10 million people who have a history of cancer are alive today.

In other words, cancer is becoming a disease that doctors can manage. To help build your sense of hope:

- Plan your days as you have always done.
- Don't limit the things you like to do just because you have cancer.
- Look for your own reasons to have hope.

Gratitude

"I do have a lot of bad days, but you know, I don't talk about those. I forget those. I think about all the good things, and I have a lot of nice times when I'm with my grandchildren, when I go to church, and when I'm with my friends." —Helen

Some people see their cancer coming back as a "wake-up call." They may realize the importance of enjoying the little things in life. They go places they've never been. They finish projects they had started but put aside. They spend more time with friends and family. They mend broken relationships.

It may be hard at first, but you can find joy in your life. Take note of what makes you smile. Pay attention to the things you do each day that you enjoy. They can be as simple as drinking your morning coffee, sitting with a pet, or talking to a friend. These small, day-to-day activities can give you comfort and pleasure.

You can also do things that are more meaningful to you. Everyone has special things, both large and small, that bring meaning to their life. For you, it may be visiting a garden in your city or town. It may be praying in a certain chapel. Or it could be playing golf or some other sport that you love. Whatever you choose, embrace the things that bring you joy when you can.

Anxiety

"I get overwhelmed a lot. There's so much to deal with right now. And I still have to deal with all the things that were going on before I got sick again. How am I going to get to the store before it closes? Has the dog been fed? What about the report that's due at work? I start to panic when I think of all the things on my plate." —Jing

Cancer takes a toll on both your body and your mind. You are coping with so much now. You may feel overwhelmed. Pain and medicines for pain can also make you feel anxious or depressed. And you may be more likely to feel this way if you have had these feelings before.

Here are some signs of anxiety:

- Feeling very tense and nervous
- Racing heartbeat
- Sweating a lot
- Trouble breathing or catching your breath
- Having a lump in your throat or a knot in your stomach
- Feeling fear.

Feeling anxious can be normal. But if it begins to disrupt your daily life, tell a member of your health care team. They can suggest someone for you to talk to. Or they can give you medicines that will help. Some of the nondrug choices for pain may work for your anxiety as well (see page 18).

"Every tomorrow has two handles. We can take hold of it with the handle of anxiety or with the handle of faith." —Henry Ward Beecher

Fear

"Honestly, I feel scared about a lot of things. Stuff I try not to think about. It comes and goes, but there always seems to be something. Even when I'm having good days, the fear is always in the back of my mind. It never goes away really." —Deena

It's normal to feel scared and worried. You may be afraid of pain or other side effects, either from the cancer or the treatment. You may worry about looking different as a result of your treatment. You may worry about taking care of your family, paying your bills, and keeping your job. You may be afraid of dying.

Signs of Depression

■ Feeling helpless or hopeless, or that life has no meaning

■ No interest in family, friends, hobbies, or things you used to enjoy

■ Loss of appetite

■ Feeling short-tempered and grouchy

■ Not being able to get certain thoughts out of your mind

■ Crying for long periods of time or many times each day

■ Thinking about hurting or killing yourself

■ Feeling "wired," having racing thoughts or panic attacks

■ Sleep problems, such as not being able to sleep, having nightmares, or sleeping too much.

It's hard to deal with the fear of so many unknowns. Some people say it helps if you know what to expect in the future. Ask your health care team questions, so you can understand more about your cancer and treatment choices. Also, update your will and other legal papers, if you haven't already done so. Then you won't have to worry about them.

Fear can be overwhelming. Remember that others have felt this way, too. It's okay to ask for help.

Sadness and Depression

"I feel sad a good bit of the time now. One thing that cheers me up is to be with my 4-year-old grandson. I love watching him as he grows more and more each day. Sometimes just thinking about him makes me feel better." —Pat

Sadness is a normal response to any serious illness. You may feel sad that you have to go through treatment again. You may feel sad that life won't be quite the same from now on.

It's okay to feel blue. You don't need to be upbeat all the time or pretend to be cheerful. Many people say that they want the freedom to just give in to their feelings sometimes. But others say that it helps to look for what is good in life, even in the bad times.

Depression can happen when sadness or despair seems to take over your life. Some of the signs listed on the next page are normal at a time like this. But if they last more than two weeks, talk to your doctor. Some symptoms could be due to physical problems. This is why it's important to let your doctor know about them.

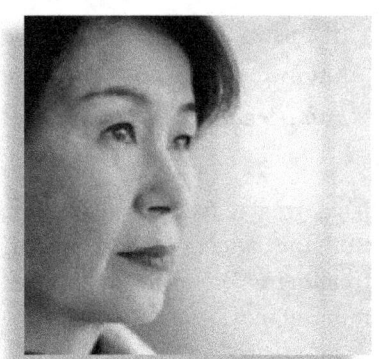

Anger

"It challenged my faith... But I've come out of it okay. It was tough in the beginning, trying to understand why this would happen to me." —Bob

You may also feel angry or frustrated. It's normal to ask, "Why me?" You may be mad at the cancer, your doctors, or your loved ones. If you are religious, you might even be angry with God. If you feel angry, it's helpful to remember that you don't have to pretend that everything is okay.

Try to figure out why you are angry. Anger sometimes comes from feelings that are hard to show. These might be fear, panic, frustration, worry, or helplessness.

It's not always easy to look at what is causing your anger. But it's healthy to try. Being open and dealing with your anger may help you let go of it. It's also good to know that anger is a form of energy. You can express this energy through exercise, art, or even just hitting the bed with a pillow.

Guilt

"I'm so tired all the time. I feel bad that my mom has to take care of me and handle things for me like she did when I was younger. I see everything she and Dad are dealing with, yet there's nothing I can do about it. I know they hate the fact that I'm going through this. I try to do what I can, but I can't stop feeling guilty for what they are going through, too." —Anne

It's normal for some people to wonder whether they did things that caused their cancer to recur. People feel guilty for a number of reasons:

- They worry about how their family and friends feel.
- They envy other people's good health and are ashamed of this feeling.
- They blame themselves for certain lifestyle choices.
- They feel guilty that their first treatment didn't work.
- They wonder if they waited too long to go back to the doctor. Or they fear that they didn't follow the doctor's instructions the right way.

But it's important to remember that the treatment failed you. *You didn't fail the treatment.* We can't know why cancer returns in some people and not others. So, it's important for you to try to:

- Focus on things worthy of your time and energy.
- Let go of any mistakes you think you may have made.
- Forgive yourself.

You may want to share these feelings with your loved ones. Some people blame themselves for upsetting the people they love or worry that they'll be a burden to others. If you feel this way, take comfort knowing that many family members say that it is an honor and a privilege to care for their loved one. Many consider it a time when they can share experiences and become closer to one another. Others say that caring for someone else makes them take life more seriously and causes them to reevaluate their priorities.

If you don't feel that you can talk openly about these things with your loved ones, getting counseling or joining a support group may also help. Let your health care team know if you would like to talk with someone about your feelings.

Loneliness

"I have lots of people around me who care, but I still feel like no one really understands." —Carlos

You may feel lonely, even when lots of people support and care for you. Here are some common feelings:

- You feel like no one else understands what you're going through, even those you love and care about.

- You feel distant from others. Or you find that your family and friends have a hard time dealing with your cancer.

- You realize that you aren't able to take part in as many events and activities as you used to.

Although it may be harder some days than others, remember that you aren't alone. Continue to do the things you've always done as best you can. If you want to, tell people that you don't want to be alone and that you welcome their visits. More than likely, your loved ones have feelings like yours. They may feel isolated from you and lonely if they are unable to talk with you.

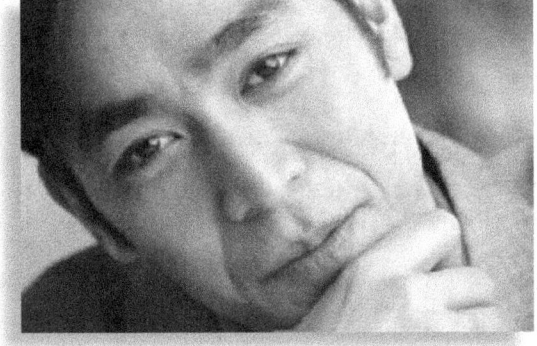

Denial

You may feel that this is not happening to you. It's tough to accept that the cancer has come back. Feeling that you need more time to absorb everything is natural. You may need more time to adjust to the news. But this can become a serious problem if it lasts longer than it should. It can keep you from getting the treatment you need or talking about your treatment choices. As time passes, try to keep an open mind. Listen to what others around you suggest for your care.

Ways You Can Cope

Your feelings will come and go, just like they always have. If you have some strategies to deal with them, you have already taken a step in the right direction.

Know that many other people have been where you are. Some do better when they join a support group. It helps them to talk with others who are facing the same challenges. You may prefer to join an online support group. That way you can chat with people from home. Be sure to check the privacy issues before you join.

If support groups don't appeal to you, there are many experts who are trained to give cancer support. These include oncology social workers, psychologists or health psychologists, counselors, or members of your faith or spiritual community. For more information, see the Resources section on page 37.

> What I need at least once or twice a week is to talk to one or a group of people who are in the same shoes as I am." —Vince

A Word About Support Groups

You may have heard about support groups in your area for people with cancer. They can meet in person, by phone, or over the Internet. They may help you gain new insights into what's happening, get ideas about how to cope, and help you know that you're not alone.

In a support group, people may talk about their feelings and what they have gone through. They may trade advice and try to help others who are dealing with the same kinds of issues. Some people like to go and just listen. Others prefer not to join support groups at all. Some people aren't comfortable with this kind of sharing.

If you feel like you would enjoy outside support such as this, but can't get to a group in your area, try a support group on the Internet. Some people with cancer say that Web sites with support groups have helped them a lot.

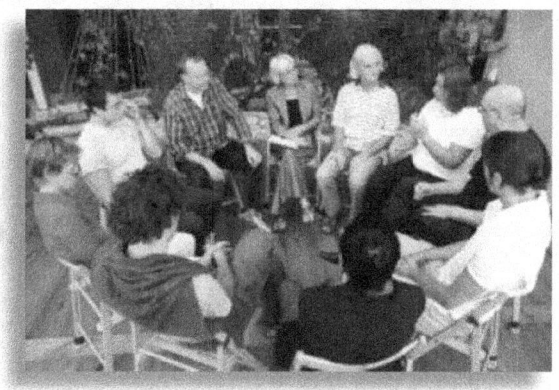

Ways You Can Cope

You may be able to continue many of your regular activities, even though some may be more difficult than before. Whatever you do, remember to conserve your strength for the things you really want to do. Don't plan too many things for one day. Also try to stagger them during the day.

Here are some things other people with cancer say have helped them cope. As you can see, even the little things help!

I built a birdhouse with my grandson. We had fun, and I loved teaching him about tools.

Spend time with the people I love.

I watch a lot of movies.

I like to fix things around the house.

I took up photography. I didn't buy a fancy camera or anything— I just started taking pictures.

I'm taking a watercolor class. I'm awful at it, but I sure don't care—anything that gets my mind off things.

I like to get my nails done.

I started to follow the stock market.

My nieces call and leave messages or songs on my answering machine. I listen to them when I need a fast way of cheering up.

Sometimes I drive out to the airport and watch the planes. For some reason, it's very soothing to me.

Build model airplanes.

Arrange flowers.

Window shop.

People watch at the mall.

Go to a movie.

Play board games or cards.

Attend local concerts and plays.

Start a new daily routine. Accept that it may have to be different from your old one— change is okay!

Talk about feelings with friends, family, or a leader in your faith or spiritual community.

Do exercise, yoga or gentle stretching.

Go fishing.

Do the things I enjoy, like making phone calls or reading.

Listen to music or a relaxation tape.

Do woodcarving.

I like to bird-watch. I sit on my porch with a pair of binoculars.

Read mystery novels.

Spend time outdoors in a community garden or park.

Volunteer or find a way to help others in need.

Plant flowers.

Go to worship services.

Knit, crochet, or do needlepoint.

Do crossword puzzles.

Meditate or do relaxation exercises.

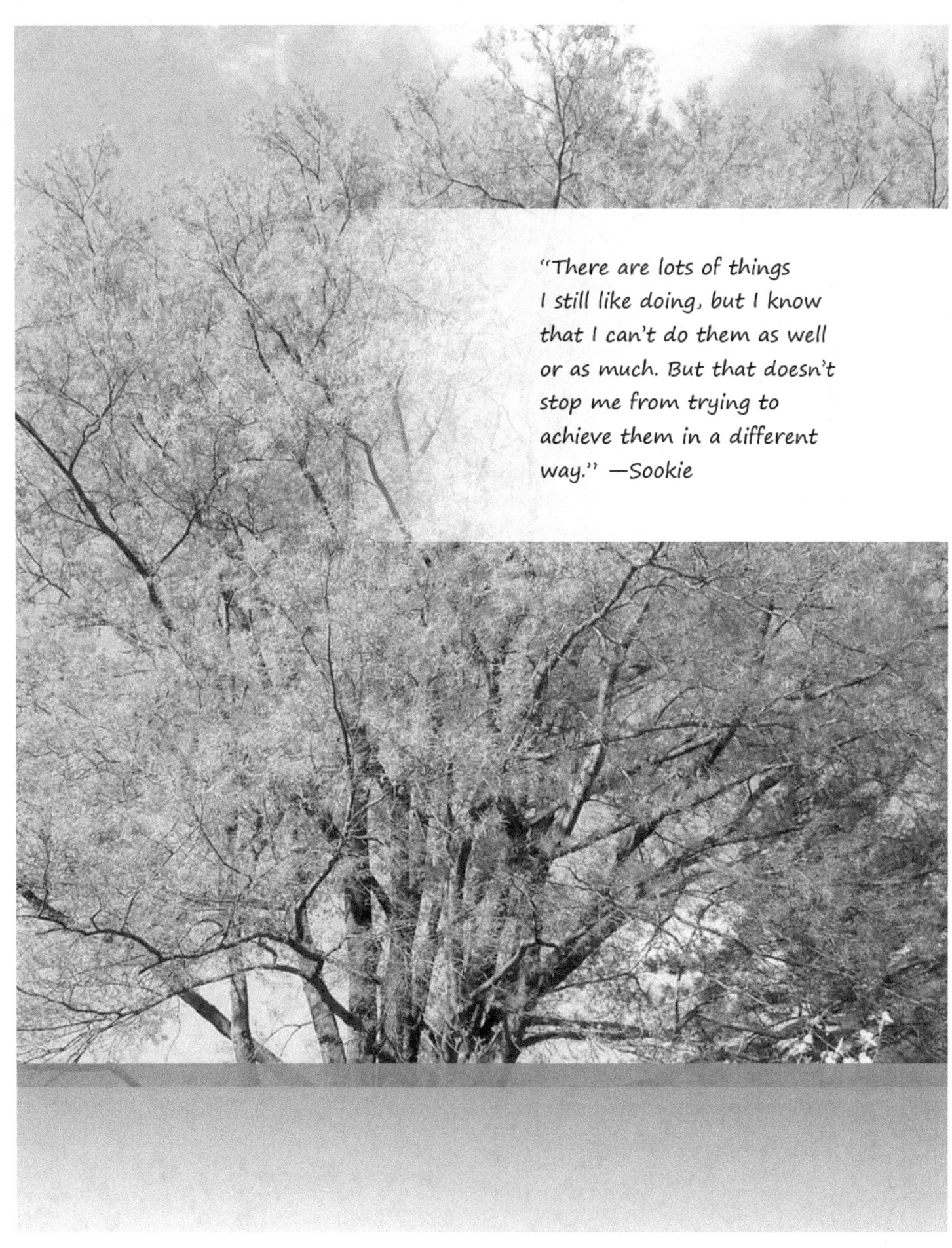

"There are lots of things I still like doing, but I know that I can't do them as well or as much. But that doesn't stop me from trying to achieve them in a different way." —Sookie

CHAPTER 6

Setting Goals

Cancer treatment can take up a lot of your time and energy. It helps to plan something that takes your mind off the disease each day. Aim for small goals each day, such as:

- Exercising

- Completing tasks you've been wanting to do

- Making phone calls

- Having lunch with a friend

- Reading one chapter of a book or doing a puzzle

- Listening to music or a relaxation tape.

Many people with cancer also set longer-term goals. They say that they do much better if they set goals or look forward to something special. It could be an anniversary, the birth of a child or grandchild, a wedding, a graduation, or a vacation. But if you set a long-term goal, make sure you are realistic about how you will achieve it.

Remember, too, that being flexible is important. You may have to change your plans if your energy level drops. You may have to adjust your goals if the cancer causes new challenges. Whatever your goals, try to spend your time in a way that you enjoy.

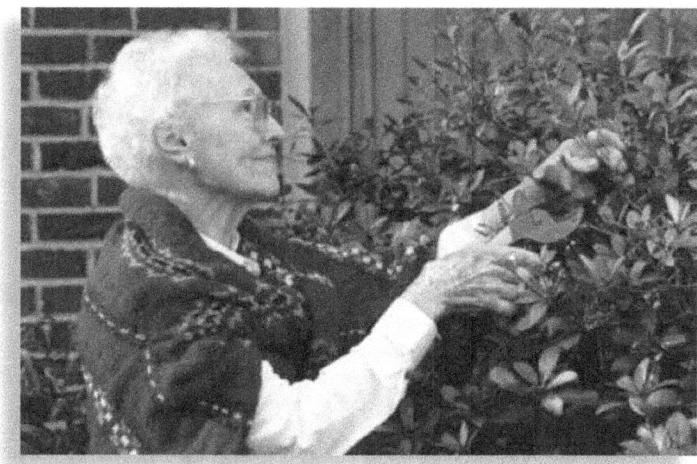

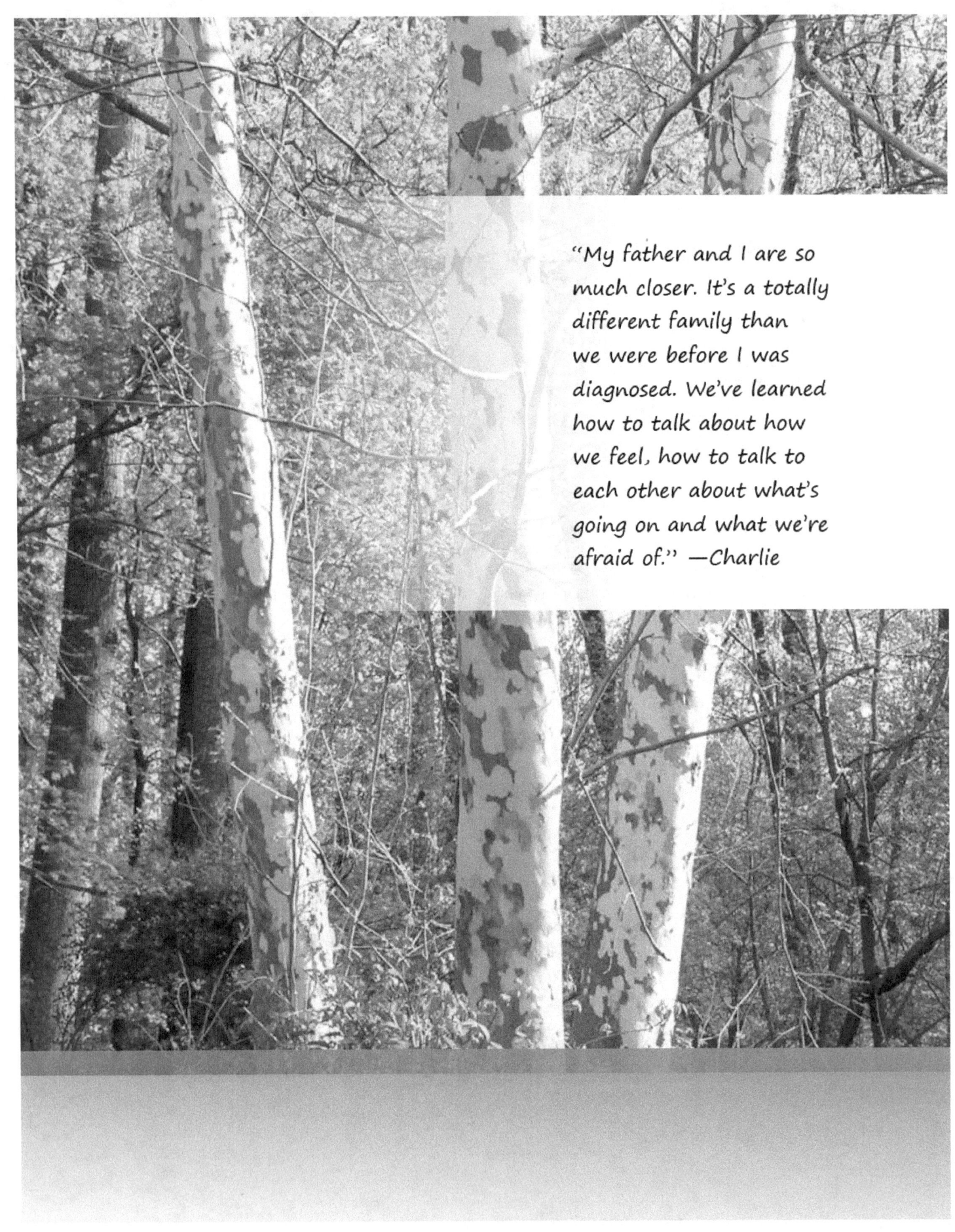

"My father and I are so much closer. It's a totally different family than we were before I was diagnosed. We've learned how to talk about how we feel, how to talk to each other about what's going on and what we're afraid of." —Charlie

CHAPTER 7

Family and Friends

Your loved ones may need time to adjust to the news that your cancer has returned. They need to come to terms with their own feelings. These may include confusion, shock, helplessness, anger, and other feelings.

Let family members and friends know that they can offer comfort just by:

- Being themselves
- Listening and not trying to solve problems
- Being at ease with you.

Knowing that they are able to comfort you may help them cope with their feelings.

Bear in mind that not everyone can handle the return of cancer. Sometimes a friend or family member can't face the idea that you might not get better. Some people may not know what to say or do for you. As a result, relationships may change, but not because of you. They may change because others can't cope with their own feelings and pain. If you can, remind your loved ones that you are still the same person you always were. Let them know if it's all right to ask questions or tell you how they feel. Sometimes just reminding them to be there for you is enough.

It's also okay if you don't feel comfortable talking about your cancer. Some topics are hard to talk about with people you are close to. In this case, you may want to talk with a member of your health care team or a trained counselor. You might want to attend a support group where people meet to share common concerns.

Family Meetings

Some families have trouble expressing their needs to each other. Other families simply do not get along. If you don't feel comfortable talking with family members, ask a member of your health care team to help. You could also ask a social worker or other professional to hold a family meeting. This may help family members feel that they can safely express their feelings. It can also be a time for you and your family to meet with your entire health care team to solve problems and set goals. Although it can be very hard to talk about these things, studies show that cancer care is a smoother process when everyone remains open and talks about the issues.

> "It's a roller coaster ride, so we just ride the roller coaster. I've got the whole family prepared, and that's what you have to do when you have cancer. Things are going well one minute, but you never know when they're going to change." —Gwen

People Close to You

Often, talking with someone close to you is harder than talking with anyone else. Here's some advice on talking with loved ones during tough times.

Spouses and Partners

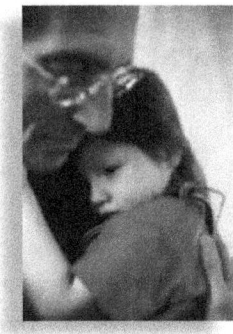

- Try as much as you can to keep your relationship as it was before you got sick.

- Talk things over. This may be hard for you or your spouse or partner. If so, ask a counselor or social worker to talk with both of you together.

- Be realistic about demands. Your spouse or partner may feel guilty about your illness. They may feel guilty about any time spent away from you. They also may be under stress due to changing family roles.

- Spend some time apart. Your spouse or partner needs time to address their own needs. If these needs are neglected, your loved one may have less energy and support to give. Remember, you didn't spend 24 hours a day together before you got sick.

- Body changes and emotional concerns may affect your sex life. Talking openly and honestly is key. But if you can't talk about these issues, you might want to talk with a professional. Don't be afraid to seek help or advice if you need it.

Children

Keeping your children's trust is very important at this time. Children can sense when things are wrong. So it's best to be as open as you can about your cancer. They may worry that they did something to cause the cancer. They may be afraid that no one will take care of them. They may also feel that you are not spending as much time with them as you used to. Although you can't protect them from what they might feel, you can prepare them for these feelings.

Some children become clingy. Others get into trouble at school or at home. It helps to keep the lines of communication open. Try to:

- Be honest. Tell them you are sick and that the doctors are working to make you better.

- Let them know that nothing they did or said caused the cancer. And make sure that they know that they can't catch it from you.

- Reassure them that you love them.

- Encourage them to talk about their feelings.

- Tell them it's okay to be upset, angry, or scared.

- Be clear and simple when you talk, since children can focus only briefly. Use words they can understand.

- Let them know they will be taken care of and loved.

- Let them know that it's okay to ask questions. Tell them that you will answer them as honestly as you can. In fact, children who aren't told the truth about an illness can become even more scared. They often depend on their imagination and fears to explain the changes around them.

Teenagers

Teenagers have some of the same needs as those of younger children. They need to hear the truth about an illness. This helps keep them from feeling needless guilt and stress. But be aware that they may try to avoid the subject. They may become angry, act out, or get into trouble as a way of coping. Others simply withdraw. Try to:

■ Give them the space they need. This is especially important if you are relying on them more to help with family needs.

■ Give them time to deal with their feelings, alone or with friends.

■ Let them know that they should still go to school and take part in sports and other fun activities.

If you have trouble explaining your cancer, you might want to ask for help. A close friend, relative, healthcare worker, or trusted coach or teacher could help answer your teenager's questions. Your support group, social worker, or doctor can also help you find a counselor or psychologist.

Adult Children

Your relationship with your adult children may change now that you have cancer again. You may have to rely on them more. And it may be hard for you to ask for support. After all, you may be used to giving support rather than getting it.

Adult children have their concerns, too. They may start to think about their own mortality. They may feel guilt, because of the many demands on them as parents, children, and employees. Some may live far away or have other duties. They may feel bad that they can't spend as much time with you as they would like. Often it helps to:

■ Share decision-making with your children.

■ Involve them in issues that are important to you. These may include treatment choices, plans for the future, or activities that you want to continue.

■ If they aren't able to be there with you, keep them updated on your progress.

■ Make the most of the time you have. Share your feelings with them.

Try to reach out to your adult children. Openly sharing your feelings, goals, and wishes will help them adjust. It will also help prevent problems in the future. Remember, just as parents want the best for their children, children want the best for their parents. They want to see your needs met effectively and with compassion. Your children don't want to see you suffer.

When a Parent Has Cancer

"My illness became a vehicle for teaching my children lessons I'd want to teach them if I'd never been sick. Instead of fighting or trying to hide all the challenges, I used them to teach my kids the value of delayed gratification, how to find hope when the chips are down, that you are the same person inside even if your appearance changes, and that you try your best and forgive yourself if things don't go well.

"My treatments became a powerful way to say to my children, 'I love you and will do whatever I must to be with you.'" —Wendy Harpham, M.D., author of *When a Parent Has Cancer: A Guide to Caring for Your Children*

"I really struggled with my diagnosis. I couldn't understand why I had to go through this one more time. Although I wouldn't consider myself religious, I found that prayer helped me. I began to feel as if I had a purpose in life, and that the cancer was just part of the plan." —Bill

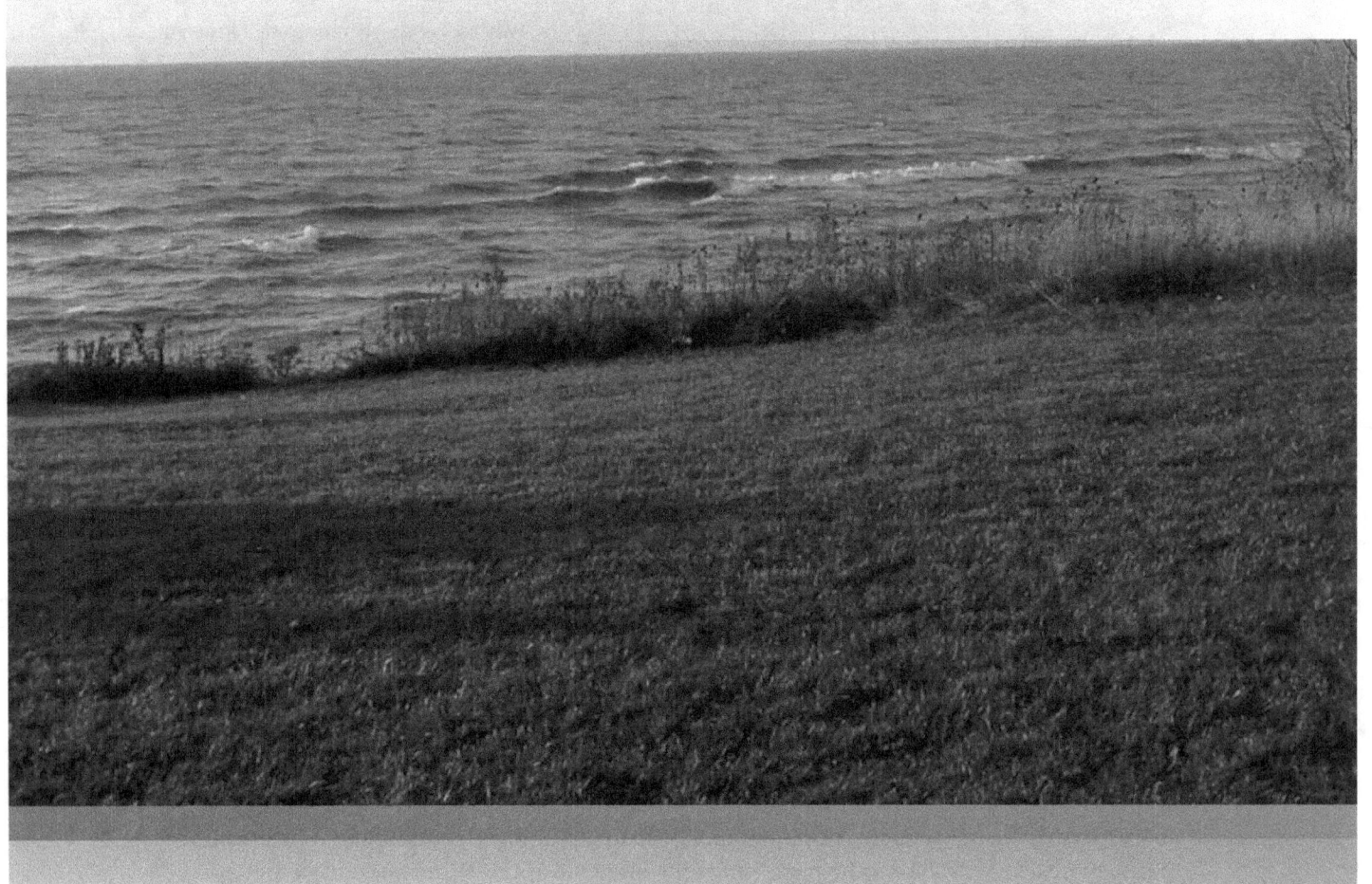

CHAPTER 8

Looking for Meaning

At different times in life, it's natural for people to look for meaning in their lives. And many people with recurrent cancer find this search for meaning important. They want to understand their purpose in life. They often reflect on what they have gone through. Some look for a sense of peace or a bond with others. Some seek to forgive themselves or others for past actions. Some look for answers and strength through religion or spirituality.

Being spiritual means different things to different people. It's a very personal issue. Everyone has their own beliefs about the meaning of life. Some people find it through religion or faith. Some find it by teaching or through volunteer work. Others find it in other ways. Having cancer may cause you to think about what you believe—about God, an afterlife, or the connections between living things. This can bring a sense of peace, a lot of questions, or both.

You may have already given a lot of thought to these issues. Still, you might find comfort by exploring more deeply what is meaningful to you. You could do this with someone close to you, a member of your faith or spiritual community, a counselor, or a trusted friend. Or you may find that talking to others at gatherings and services at places of worship is helpful.

Or you may just want to take time for yourself. You may want to reflect on your experiences and relationships. Writing in a journal or reading also helps some people find comfort and meaning. Others find that prayer or meditation helps them.

Many people also find that cancer changes their values. The things you own and your daily duties may seem less important. You may decide to spend more time with loved ones or helping others. You may want to do more things outdoors or learn something new.

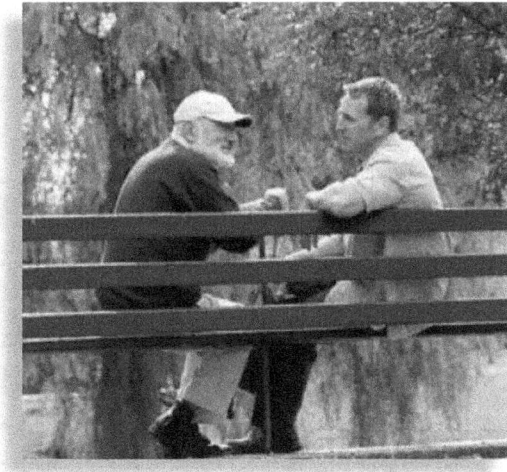

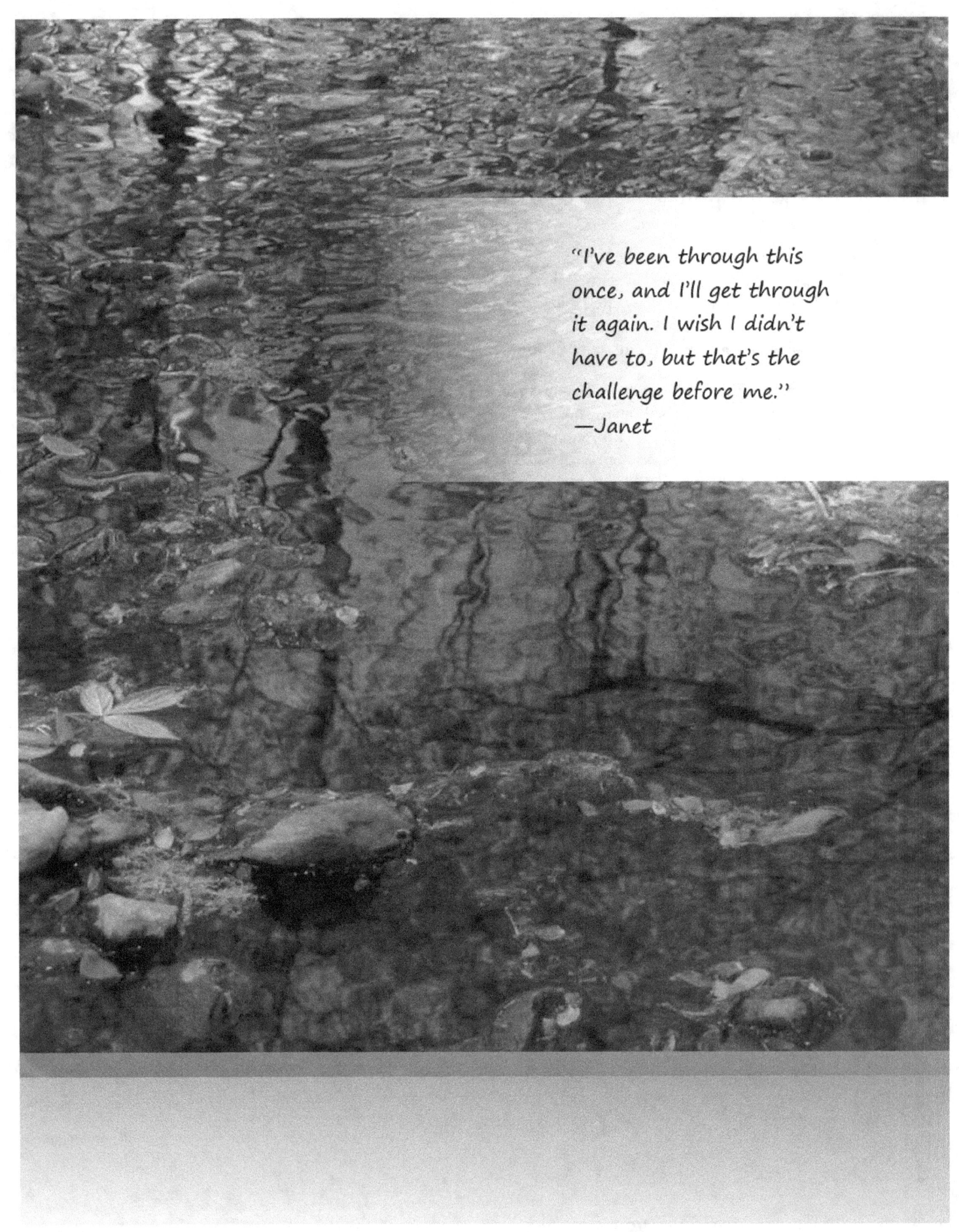

"I've been through this once, and I'll get through it again. I wish I didn't have to, but that's the challenge before me."
—Janet

CHAPTER 9

A Time To Reflect

This is a hard time in your life. Living with cancer is tough, especially when it has come back. You battled the disease once, and now you must face it again. But you're more experienced this time around.

Use this knowledge to your advantage. Try to remember what you did before to cope. Reflect on what you might have done differently. By looking back in this way, the hope is that you may find new strength. And that this strength can help carry you through each day, and through the coming weeks and months.

"Think only of today,

and when tomorrow comes,

it will be today,

and we will think about it."

—St. Francis de Sales

Words To Know

Acupuncture (AK-yoo-PUNK-cher): A form of Chinese medicine that stimulates certain points on the body. It is often done using thin needles. Before using acupuncture, ask your health care team if it is safe for your type of cancer.

Advance directives: Legal documents that allow you to decide ahead of time how you want to be treated when you are unable to speak for yourself. The two main types are living wills and durable power of attorney for health care.

Biofeedback: Using a special machine, a person learns how to control certain body functions. Examples of such body functions are heart rate and blood pressure.

Biological (bye-uh-LAHJ-uh-kul) **therapy**: Treatment that aims to use or restore the body's own immune (defense) system. It is used to fight cancer, infections, and other diseases. It is also used to reduce the side effects that some cancer treatments cause. Also called immunotherapy.

Breakthrough pain: Pain that is sudden and intense or that is very painful for a short time. It can occur several times a day. This can happen even when a person is taking the right dose of pain medicine.

Cancer: A term for diseases in which abnormal cells divide out of control. Cancer cells can invade nearby tissues and spread through the bloodstream and lymphatic system to other parts of the body.

Chemotherapy (kee-moh-THAIR-uh-pee): Treatment with drugs that kill cancer cells.

Clinical trial: A type of research study that tests new methods of screening, prevention, treatment, or diagnosis of a disease. Also called a clinical study.

Complementary and alternative medicine (CAM): Treatment used along with, or instead of, standard health care. CAM includes methods such as acupuncture and massage. Some CAM treatments may help relieve cancer symptoms or side effects. But not all CAM treatments are safe. And they should not take the place of standard health care.

Diagnosis (dye-ug-NOH-sis): The name and details of your disease or health condition.

Dietitian (dy-uh-TIH-sun): A person with special training in nutrition, who can help you with choices in your diet. They also can suggest ways to make eating easier.

Distant cancer: Cancer that has spread from the primary tumor to distant organs or lymph nodes.

Durable power of attorney for health care: This type of advance directive appoints a person (a health care proxy) to make medical decisions for you when you can't make them for yourself.

Health care proxy: The person you have named in an advance directive to make medical decisions for you. This person can make health care choices for you when you can't make them for yourself.

Health psychologist: A mental health professional who works with people and families affected by illness.

Hypnosis: A state of relaxed and focused attention. The person focuses on a certain feeling, idea, or suggestion.

Imagery: A method in which a person focuses on positive images in their mind.

I.V.: Short for intravenous (in-truh-VEE-nus). It means to get medicine or nutrients into the body through a vein.

Living will: A type of advance directive. A living will is a legal document that lets people know what kind of medical care you want if you are unable to speak for yourself.

Local cancer: Cancer that appears only in the organ where the cancer began. It has not spread beyond the original site.

Lymph (limf) **nodes:** Small, bean-shaped organs that are part of the lymphatic system. Bacteria or cancer cells that enter the lymphatic system may be found in the nodes. Also called lymph glands.

Massage therapy: Gentle rubbing of different body parts or muscles to help you relax and gain a sense of well-being.

Metastasis (meh-TASS-tuh-sis): The spread of cancer from one part of the body to another. Cells that have metastasized are like those in the original tumor.

Notary public: A person with authority from the courts to witness legal documents and signatures.

Oncologist (ahn-KAH-luh-jist): A doctor who specializes in treating cancer.

Oncology social worker: A social worker who specializes in helping cancer patients and their families.

Palliative (PAL-ee-yuh-tiv) **care:** Care to improve the quality of life of people with a serious or life-threatening illness. The goal of palliative care is to prevent or treat as early as possible:
- Symptoms of the disease
- Side effects caused by treatment
- Psychological, social, and spiritual problems related to the disease or its treatment.

Also called comfort care, supportive care, and symptom management.

Power of attorney: Appoints a person to make financial decisions for you when you can't make them yourself.

Radiation (ray-dee-AY-shun) **therapy**: Treatment with high-energy radiation to kill cancer cells.

Recurrence (ree-KUR-ens): Cancer that has come back after a period of time during which it could not be found. The cancer may come back to the same place as the original tumor or to another place in the body. Also called recurrent cancer.

Recurrent cancer: See "recurrence."

Regional cancer: Cancer that has grown beyond the original tumor to nearby lymph nodes or organs and tissues.

Relaxation techniques: Different methods, such as deep breathing and relaxing the muscles, that are used to reduce tension and anxiety and to control pain.

Second opinion: When you go to another doctor after getting a diagnosis. The second doctor looks at your test results and examines you, just as the first one did. The second doctor may or may not make the same diagnosis. And they may or may not recommend the same treatment. Either way, you will have more information. This may help you decide on your treatment.

Specialist: A doctor who has studied and trained in a certain area of medicine.

Standard treatment: In medicine, treatment that experts agree is appropriate, accepted, and widely used. Also called standard of care or best practice.

Surgery (SER-juh-ree): A medical procedure that involves entering or cutting into the body. Surgery is used to remove or repair a part of the body or to find out whether disease is present.

Trust: This type of legal document appoints a person you choose to manage your money for you .

Tumor (TOO-mur): An abnormal mass of tissue.

Will: This type of legal document tells how you want to divide your money and property among your heirs.

Resources

Federal Resources

For more resources:

See *National Organizations That Offer Cancer-Related Services* at www.cancer.gov. In the search box, type in the words "national organizations."

Or call 1-800-4-CANCER (1-800-422-6237) to seek more help.

National Cancer Institute

Provides current information on cancer prevention, screening, diagnosis, treatment, genetics, and supportive care. Lists clinical trials and specific cancer topics in NCI's Physician Data Query (PDQ®) database.

Visit: www.cancer.gov

Cancer Information Service

Answers questions about cancer, clinical trials, and cancer-related services and helps users find information on the NCI Web site. Provides NCI printed materials.

Toll-free: 1-800-4-CANCER (1-800-422-6237)

Visit: www.cancer.gov/cis

Chat online: Click on "LiveHelp."

Administration on Aging

Provides information, assistance, individual counseling, organization of support groups, caregiver training, respite care, and supplemental services.

Phone: 1-202-619-0724

Visit: www.aoa.gov

Centers for Medicare and Medicaid Services

Provides information for consumers about patient rights, prescription drugs, and health insurance issues, including Medicare and Medicaid.

Toll-free: 1-800-MEDICARE (1-800-633-4227)

Visit: www.medicare.gov (for Medicare information) or
www.cms.hhs.gov (other information)

Equal Employment Opportunity Commission

Provides fact sheets about job discrimination, protections under the Americans With Disabilities Act, and employer responsibilities. Coordinates investigations of employment discrimination.

Toll-free: 1-800-669-4000

TTY: 1-800-669-6820

Visit: www.eeoc.gov

■ **U.S. Department of Labor Office of Disability Employment Policy**
Provides fact sheets on a variety of disability issues, including discrimination, workplace accommodation, and legal rights.

Phone: 1-866-633-7365

TTY: 1-877-889-5627

Visit: www.dol.gov/odep/

Private/NonProfit Organizations

■ **American Cancer Society**
National Cancer Information Center
Available to answer questions 24 hours a day, 7 days a week.

Toll-free: 1-800-ACS-2345 (1-800-227-2345)

Visit: www.cancer.org

■ **CancerCare**
Offers free support, information, financial assistance, and practical help to people with cancer and their loved ones.

Toll-free: 1-800-813-HOPE (1-800-813-4673)

Visit: www.cancercare.org

■ **Cancer Support Community**
Cancer Support Community is a national organization that provides support groups, stress reduction and cancer education workshops, nutrition guidance, exercise sessions, and social events.

Phone: 1-888-793-WELL (1-888-793-9355)

Visit: www.cancersupportcommunity.org

■ **Kids Konnected**
Offers education and support for children who have a parent with cancer or who have lost a parent to cancer.

Toll-free: 1-800-899-2866

Visit: www.kidskonnected.org

Lance Armstrong Foundation

The Lance Armstrong Foundation seeks to inspire and empower people living with, through, and beyond cancer to live strong. It provides education, advocacy, and public health and research programs.

Phone: 1-512-236-8820 (general number)

                1-866-235-7205 (LIVESTRONG SurvivorCare program)

Web site: www.livestrong.org

National Coalition for Cancer Survivorship

Provides information on cancer support, employment, financial and legal issues, advocacy, and related issues.

Phone: 1-877-NCCS YES (1-877-622-7937)

Visit: www.canceradvocacy.org

National Employment Lawyers Association

Can help find a lawyer experienced in job discrimination cases.

Phone: 1-415-296-7629

Visit: www.nela.org

NeedyMeds—Indigent Patient Programs

Lists medicine assistance programs available from drug companies.
NOTE: Usually patients cannot apply directly to these programs. Ask your doctor, nurse, or social worker to contact them.

Visit: www.needymeds.com

Patient Advocate Foundation

Offers education, legal counseling, and referrals concerning managed care, insurance, financial issues, job discrimination, and debt crisis matters.

Toll-free: 1-800-532-5274

Visit: www.patientadvocate.org

Notes